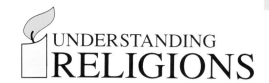

UNDERSTANDING
RELIGIONS

Birth Customs

Lucy Rushton

Wayland

Understanding Religions

Birth Customs
Death Customs
Food and Fasting
Initiation Customs
Marriage Customs
Pilgrimages and Journeys

About this book

This book looks at many customs associated with birth in the six major religions around the world. Looking at what people do and say at the most important times of their lives can help us to understand their religions. The birth of a baby is one of the times when people show what they believe in and care about.

As well as describing different practices, **Birth Customs** provides an introduction to the principles and beliefs behind these practices. Each chapter deals with one theme associated with birth, across the religions, so that readers may compare different attitudes and beliefs closely. Basic beliefs, such as having one life on earth, or being reborn, are introduced to explain different reactions to the birth of a child.

The quotations in the book will encourage children to look at the religious practices of their own communities. Teachers will find that elements of each chapter can be used as starting points for project work.

Editor: Joanna Housley
Designer: Malcolm Walker

First published in 1992 by
Wayland (Publishers) Limited
61 Western Road, Hove
East Sussex, BN3 1JD, England

British Library Cataloguing in Publication Data
Rushton, Lucy
    Birth Customs. (Understanding Religions Series)
    I. Title II. Series
    291.4

ISBN 0 7502 0418 4

Typeset by Kudos Editorial and Design Services
Printed in Italy by G Canale C.S.p.A. Turin
Bound in Belgium by Casterman S.A.

Contents

Words that appear in **bold** in the text are explained in the glossary on page 30.

Introduction

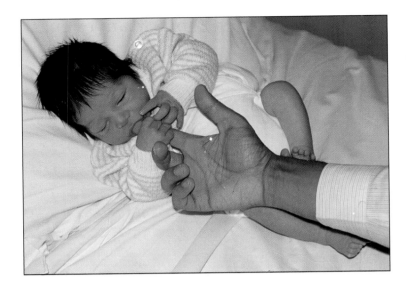

Left Already this two-day-old baby can hold firmly to its father's finger.

If you have been lucky enough to see a new-born baby you may have thought how complicated and perfect it looks. It can clutch with its tiny fingers and stare at you with dark, shiny eyes. Miraculously, it knows how to breathe and suck from the moment it is born. Even though we know so much now about how a baby grows, from a tiny speck nine months before it is born, it still seems a wonderful process.

What is your earliest memory? Can you remember anything that happened to you before you were two? Have your parents ever told you any stories about when you were a baby? Do you know if there was a special **ceremony** to mark your arrival? In many religions there are

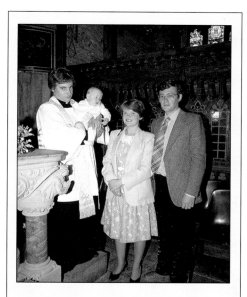

Joseph, now aged nine:
'I'm glad I was **christened** when I was a baby. If you're christened when you're a baby you can spend more of your life being a Christian. A christening means inviting the baby into God's family. You don't understand at first. It's mainly for parents and relations to remember and they tell the baby that he's been christened. As you grow older you learn about it.'

Right These candles, in a Christian cathedral, have been lit to ask God to remember somebody.

ceremonies for when a baby is born, even though the baby won't understand or remember them. Relatives and friends have ways of showing that the birth of a baby is a happy and important event.

Symbols

People use words and symbols to show what a new life means to them. A symbol can be an action or a thing which has a special meaning. A symbol to do with birth may be shaving a baby's hair, or lighting a candle. Symbols help us to think about things we find difficult to put into words.

When we read and write about people's religious beliefs and practices we need a word to represent who these practices are directed towards. People find it difficult to understand what God is like, so the word 'God' is used as a

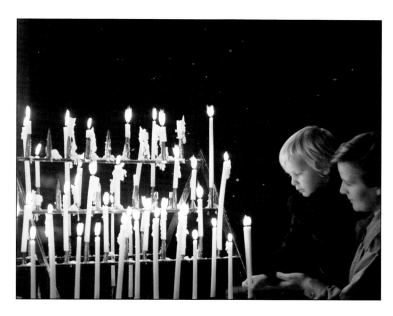

symbol. People of different **faiths** use different words for God. English-speaking Christians say God. The Jewish word is Yahweh. The Muslim word is Allah. The Sikh word is Nam. Hindus call the great spirit of their religion Brahman.

A good life

If somebody asked you what a good life is, what would you say? Followers of each religion have an idea of what makes a good life. Parents try to help their children by passing on what they themselves have found helpful and important.

Some religions teach that a person has only one life on earth. Jews, Christians and Muslims believe they have to make the most of their one life. They believe that God cares about every single person. Each new-born baby needs to be brought up as one of God's children.

Hindus, Buddhists and Sikhs all believe that part of a person, which can be called the **soul**, is born over and over again in different lives. They hope they will not be reborn on earth lots of times because they believe there is something better than life on earth.

Hindus believe that human souls came from Brahman and that Brahman is in everything in the universe. They hope that, after a long journey through many

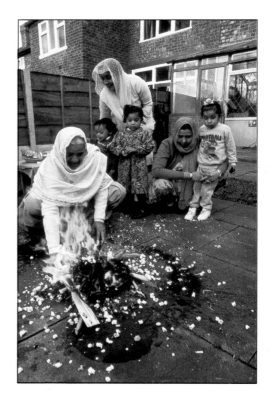

Above Most families are happy and grateful when a child is born. These Sikh women have been throwing sweets onto a fire as part of a ceremony to celebrate being able to have children. The woman in the picture has performed the ceremony many times, and is always careful not to burn her fingers.

lives, their souls will go back to Brahman. Each birth is a step on the way.

Sikh parents believe that the soul of their baby has come from God. They hope the soul will return to God after death, if the person has led a good life.

Buddhists hope to come to the end of being reborn over and over again. They hope to reach the final state of being that they call **nirvana**. You might think that Buddhists see birth as a sad event, because they want to stop being reborn. But they are happy when a baby is born, because only a human has the kind of mind which can learn to reach nirvana.

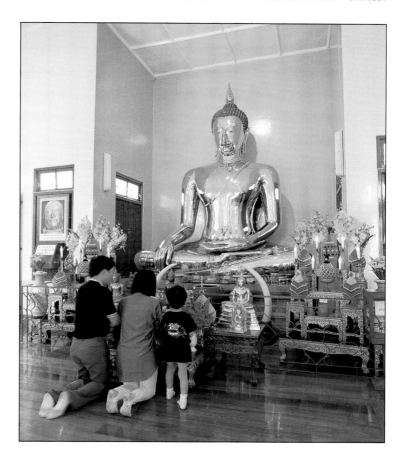

Right Buddhists respect the Buddha because they believe he discovered how to lead a life which does not lead to rebirth. This family in Thailand bring gifts of flowers and **incense** because they are grateful for the Buddha's example.

Welcome!

Waiting for a baby is usually exciting for the parents and family. They wonder whether it will be a boy or a girl and who it will look like. As the time draws near, parents make sure they have all that the baby will need. There is often a little anxiety until a baby has arrived safely. So, once the baby is born, most families celebrate to show how happy they are, and to welcome their new member.

Many parents who belong to a

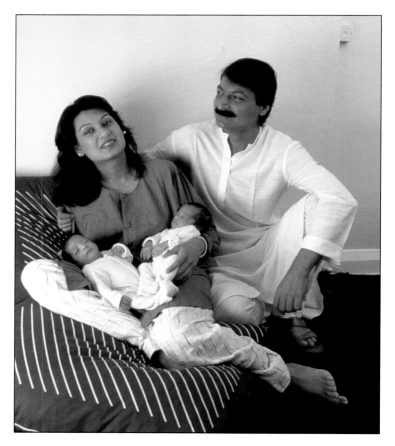

Left Parents cannot tell what will happen when they start the long wait for a baby. The birth of twins gives them twice as much to celebrate.

Shireen, a Sikh girl, says:

'After my sister was born my parents took flour, butter and sugar to the gurdwara to make the *kara parshad* for everybody, like they are doing in this temple. At home we hung leaves and money in the windows because we were celebrating.'

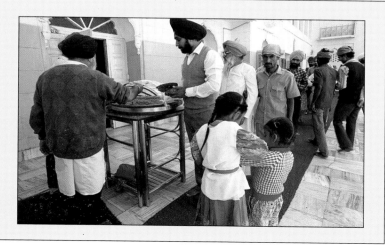

religious tradition want their baby to be welcomed into that tradition. They want their child to learn to respect their beliefs, and grow up as a member of their religious community.

Do you like sweet things? Most babies and young children like sweet things, and in many religions giving a baby something sweet to taste is a way of saying welcome. Some parents introduce a new baby to their religion by saying special words, and then giving the child something sweet to taste.

Sikh parents try to make sure that the first words their baby hears are:

*'There is one God, **Eternal** truth is His name; He made everything and is in everything. He is not afraid of anything and is not fighting anything; He is not affected by time; He was not born, He made Himself; we know about Him from the teachings of the Guru.'*

This is called the *Mool Mantra*. After

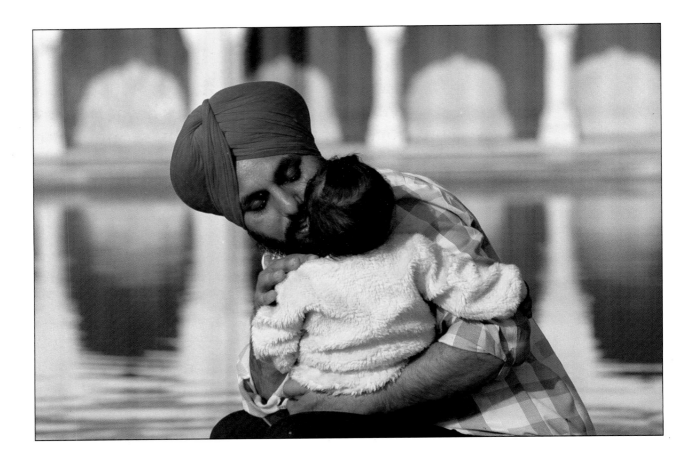

these words have been said, honey is put on the baby's tongue.

A few weeks later the baby is welcomed into the community of Sikhs. The parents take flour, butter and sugar with them when they take the child to the temple, which is called the **gurdwara**, for the first time. The flour, butter and sugar are made into a special pudding called *kara parshad*, which is shared with everyone in the temple. The baby is given a little sugary water, called *amrit*. Water is used as a symbol of purity. Sugar is a symbol of sweetness and goodness.

Above Sikh families take their children to the gurdwara from a very early age. This father and baby are outside a Sikh temple in Delhi, India.

Muslims also give new babies something sweet to taste. If a baby is born in hospital, the family hold a ceremony when it arrives home. Honey or sugar is put on the baby's tongue and a prayer is said. The meat at the *Aqiqah* (name-giving) feast may be cooked with sugar. Muslims say it makes the child sweet-tempered.

Hindus wash a new baby and then write a special word, *AUM* or *OM*, on its tongue with a golden pen dipped in honey. The word has many meanings. Hindus believe Brahman, the god of the universe, works on earth through a number of different gods. *AUM* stands for the names of the three important Hindu gods: Vishnu, Shiva and Brahma. Hindus say this word very carefully over and over again when they are praying.

Right The Hindu sacred syllable *AUM*, which is written on a baby's tongue with honey.

Belonging

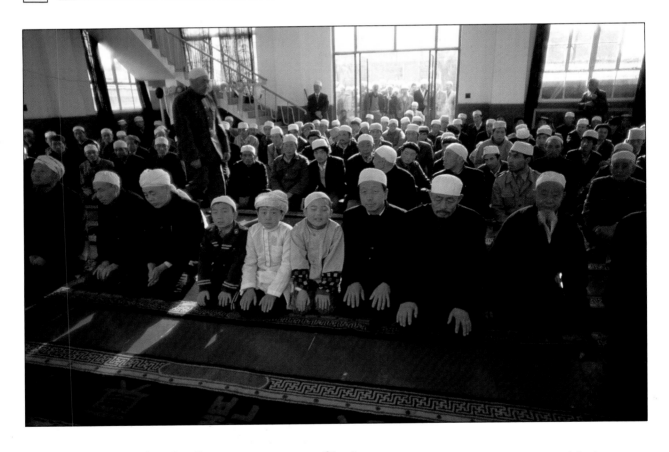

When people belong to a religious community it is like being part of a very large family. They usually have a building where they go to worship together – Jews go to a synagogue, Hindus and Buddhists to temples, Sikhs to a gurdwara, Christians to a church, and Muslims to a mosque. The people who go regularly to each place of worship see each other often and help each other if they can. Usually, parents will bring their new-born baby to meet

Above Muslims worship in a mosque. Every Friday the men go to the mosque at midday for communal prayers. Women may go too, but they remain in a different part of the mosque.

Daniel, aged nine:

'I think it is important for families to have children because Jews believe there's something inside people that goes on in other people. You grow up and have children and a bit of you is in them. Something comes to you from your parents and **ancestors**. We have a close family, and celebrate all important events together.'

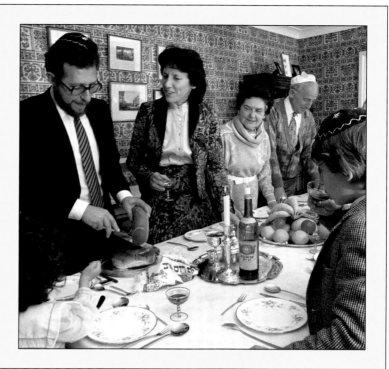

the people who go to the same place of worship and share their joy.

Jews think of themselves as part of a community that has grown up over thousands of years. They believe they have a duty to behave in a way that they think God wants them to behave, and to be an example to others. By living a good life a person can show how fair and good God is.

When a Jewish boy is born, he is **circumcised** to show that he is a member of the Jewish faith. This means that a small piece of skin is cut from the baby boy's **penis**. In **Orthodox Judaism** this is carried out at a ceremony called *Brit Milah*, when the boy is eight days old.

During the operation the boy's father says this prayer:

'Blessed are you, Lord our God, King of the Universe, who blessed us with His commandment, and ordered us to enter my son into the promise made by Abraham. As he has been entered into this promise so may he study the **Torah***, marry so that he has Your blessing, and live a good life.'*

The ceremony ends with a prayer of blessing called *kiddush* which Jews say on many occasions. Everybody drinks wine when this prayer is said, and the baby is given some to taste. The boy's name is chosen, then the men and boys go back to the rest of the family for a party.

Sometimes children are not expected to become followers of a religion until they are old enough to choose for themselves. Buddhists say that a child has to decide for him or herself that the Buddha's teaching is the right path to follow. But a Buddhist child may still be brought up in the Buddhist way of life from birth. There are Buddhist ceremonies which welcome a baby. Often **monks** come to the house to chant and bless the child. In one branch of Buddhism, sacred threads are tied around the baby's wrists when it is one month old. These threads are believed to welcome a spirit called *khwan*, which looks after the baby.

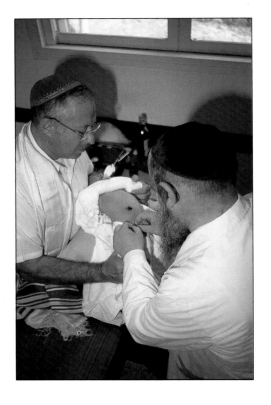

Above This new-born Jewish baby is being held by his grandfather. The man who performs the circumcision is called a *mohel*.

Like Buddhists, some Christians, called Baptists, feel that people have to decide for themselves to make a commitment of faith. They do not **baptize** babies, but have another ceremony called Dedication of Children. This takes place at a service with hymns and prayers in a church. When the child has grown up she or he can decide to be baptized and join the Church.

Right In Buddhist countries like Thailand and Burma many young boys spend some time living the simple life of a monk. Living as a monk means this Burmese boy learns what the Buddha taught in a practical way.

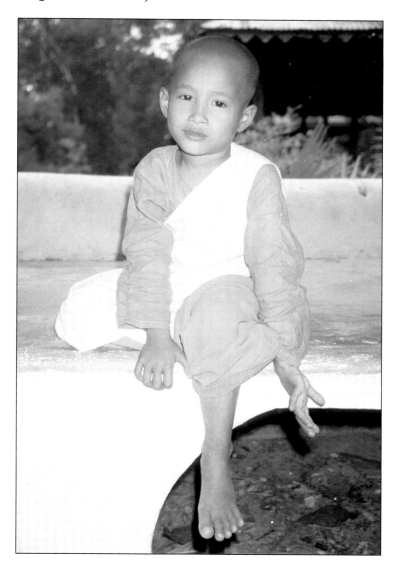

Choosing a name

Your name is something you take with you everywhere you go. For some people a name is like a membership badge, given at the time they join the community of believers. Some names have a special religious meaning and can remind people of what they believe in.

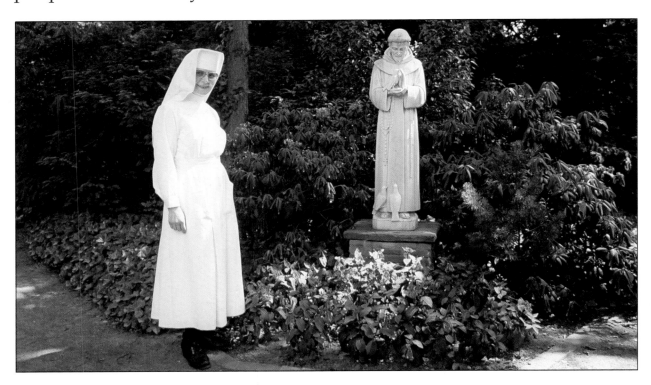

Saints

Many **Orthodox Christians** and Roman Catholics are named after saints. Saints are people who let God work in their lives. Christians believe the saints are with God after they die. Catholics and

Above This statue is of St Francis. He was a rich man who gave up everything to care for other people and all living creatures. Many Christians, like this nun, try to follow his example.

Orthodox Christians sometimes pray to saints to ask for help. They believe the saints can bring them strength from God.

Each saint has a special feast day in the year. Most Orthodox Christians and Catholics celebrate the day belonging to the saint whose name they share. It is called the name-day.

For example:

Anthony	17 January
Maria	15 August
Catherine	25 November
Nicholas	6 December

In Greece it is the custom, on a person's name-day, for all friends and relations to visit the house for a party. If you know many people with the same name you may have to make several visits!

Muslims sometimes take names from

Teresa, a Catholic, aged 8.
'A lot of Catholics are named after saints. I am named after St Theresa who was a Spanish nun. My name day is 15 October. As well as having a birthday party every year, I also have a party on my name day. It's like having two birthdays!'

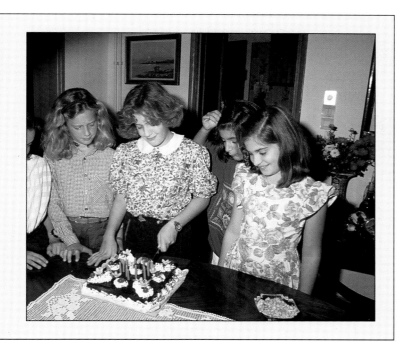

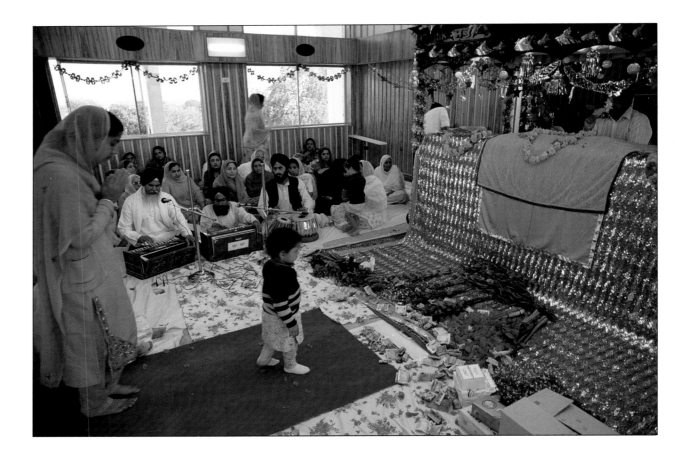

the family of Muhammad. Muhammad was the Prophet, or Messenger, of Allah. Some Muslims ask their leader (called the **imam**) to choose their child's name. He chooses names with a meaning to remind Muslims of their faith. For example, Abdullah means servant of Allah and Fardose means Heaven.

Sikh babies are named when they are taken to the gurdwara for the first time. There is a reading from the Granth, the holy book of Sikhism. The reader opens the book and looks at the first letter on the page. A name beginning with that letter is then chosen for the baby.

Above In a gurdwara the Granth is placed on a platform beneath a canopy, like the one on the right. The reader is sitting behind, facing the people.

The gift of life

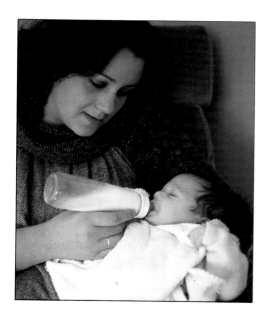

Above If a baby is loved and cared for it will learn to care for others.

People who believe in God often say the birth of a baby is one way they can see His power at work. They see that a human life is something very precious. A baby will, if cared for, grow into a lovable and loving person. That person will be someone who is able to tell right from wrong, who can care for others and try to lead a good life.

Thanking God

One way in which Muslims thank God for a baby is to give gifts to those in need. Muslims believe there are five rules in life that must be obeyed. Giving to people in need is one of these rules. It is called *zakat*.

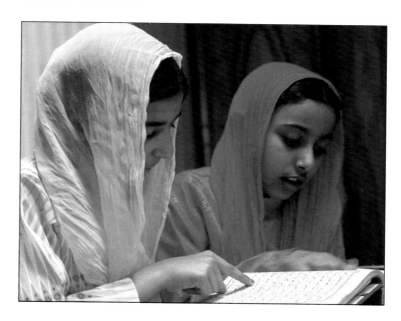

Right Muslims believe that Allah has given them the Qur'an, their holy book, to teach them how to live.

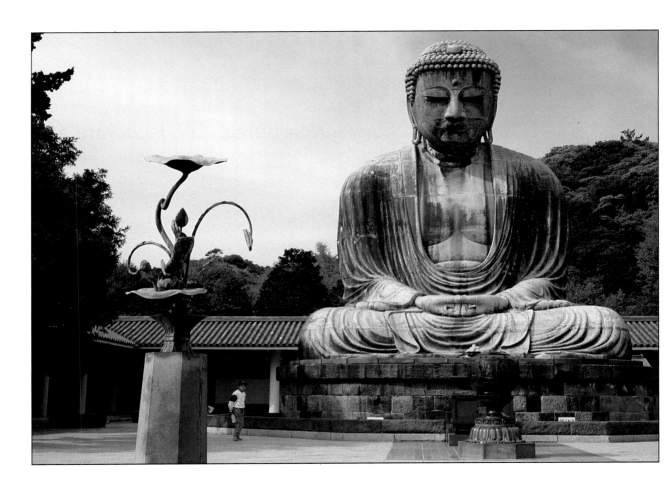

Soon after a Muslim baby has been born its hair is shaved for the name-giving ceremony. It is the custom to give away the same amount of silver as the weight of hair. Of course, hair does not weigh very much and usually the parents would give more than that. After the name-giving ceremony the family hold a feast. In Muslim countries, if the baby is a boy they kill two goats for the feast. If it is a girl they kill one. They invite friends and neighbours to share the meat, but one third of it should be given to the poor.

Above **Meditation** means calmly paying attention to your thoughts and feelings. Buddhists believe that meditation can lead to clear understanding and, in the end, to nirvana.

Buddhists believe that only humans can learn to reach the perfect state of being called nirvana. The Buddha told his followers that the chance of being born into a human life is as rare as a blind turtle putting his head up through the hole of an ox-yoke floating on the surface of the oceans. This encourages Buddhists to think of their human life as a special opportunity.

Jews read in the Torah that their ancestor, Abraham, was told by God to 'be fruitful and multiply'. They take this to mean that Jewish couples should have children, so that the community of Jews does not die out.

Below The Torah is the Jews' holy book, their guide to a good and wise life. Parents encourage their children to study it.

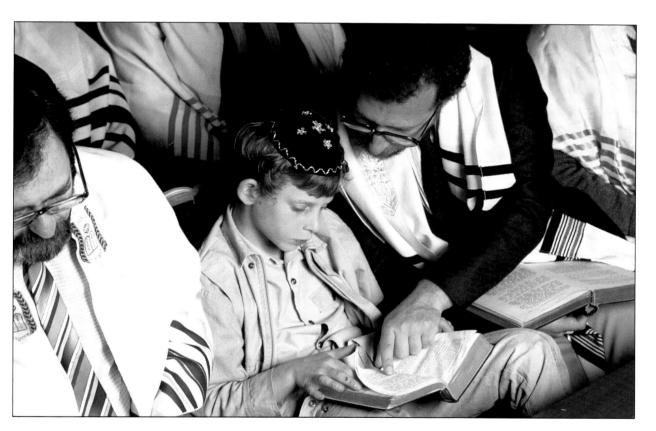

A fresh start

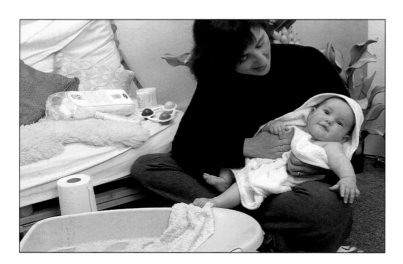

Left This baby is nice and clean after her bath. Some birth customs involve washing as a symbol for a clean start in life.

Most religions have some ceremonies for a new baby which are to do with being clean. Babies are washed in a special way, or shaved or given new clothes. These actions **symbolize** the fresh beginning of a new life.

Anybody who has a baby brother or sister knows that it is quite hard work to keep a baby clean. But that is not the main reason for these symbolic actions. Parents want their children to have the best chance in life, and being clean is a symbol for having a fresh start. It doesn't only mean having a clean body but having good thoughts and kind feelings too.

Muslims wash themselves in a special way before they pray or read the Qur'an, the Muslim holy book. Soon after a

Muslim baby is born, probably on the seventh day, they prepare it for the *Aqiqah* name-giving ceremony, by washing it and shaving its head. Like Jews, Muslims circumcise boy babies. This is done because they believe it is cleaner.

Sometimes dirt is a symbol for sins. Sins are bad ideas and actions that lead people away from their beliefs and make them forget what is important.

Salam, a Muslim girl, explains her idea of sin:

'You might be nice to someone but all the time you are thinking what you really want to do is hit her. You have to be nice inside...Allah sees what you are like inside.'

Beatrice, who is a Catholic, adds:

'Yes, you have to be pure, pure in your heart.'

Muslims and Christians agree that just because you cannot always see sin,

Right Before starting to pray, this Muslim has washed his hands, face and feet. Washing takes away dirt but also helps him to concentrate on his prayers.

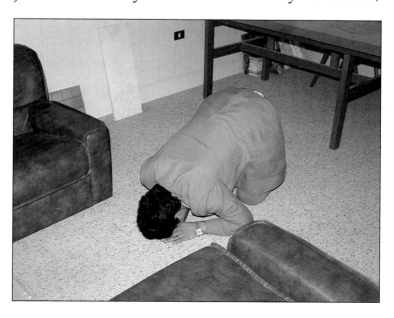

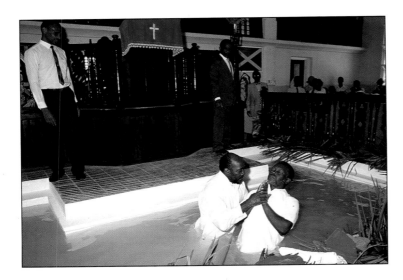

Left Some Christians baptize by putting the person completely under water. They say that coming out from the water is like being born again.

this does not mean it is not there, spoiling a person's life.

Christians believe that humans are born with sin. They believe that Jesus Christ is the son of God, and that they can be saved from sin if they follow his teachings. Baptism is a Christian symbol for washing away this natural sin so that a person can start again. Some Christians talk about baptism as a 'second birth'. When a baby is to be baptized, the child's parents choose people to be godparents. Although godparents do not look after their godchildren by feeding or clothing them, they promise to look after their other needs - the needs of their souls. They have to say during the baptism service that they reject the **devil** and trust Jesus. In the Anglican Church, godparents promise to bring the child for the ceremony of **confirmation** when he or she is old enough.

The washing which takes place at a Christian baptism is done in many different ways. Sometimes Christians go to a river to be baptized, in the way Jesus was baptized. Baptists have deep pools in their churches. Some Christians have a basin called a font in their churches. Orthodox babies are dipped completely under water three times. Roman Catholics and Anglicans pour just a little water on to the baby's forehead and mark a cross.

There is a ceremony for a Hindu child when it is one year old. The baby's head is completely shaved. Hindus believe that a person's soul goes through many lives. They want any evil from the child's past lives to be removed so that it can have a good start. The shaving of the hair is a symbol for removing any sin of past lives.

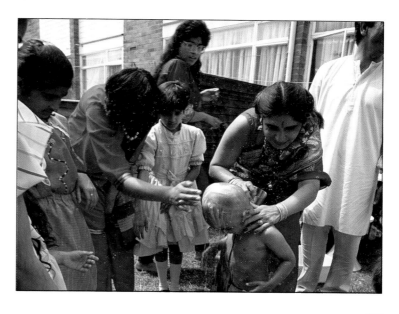

Right The family gathers round while this Hindu child's head is shaved.

The path of life

We can think of a person's life being rather like a journey. We all travel from birth to death but many events can happen in between.

Signposts
People who have a religious faith believe they are not just wandering along

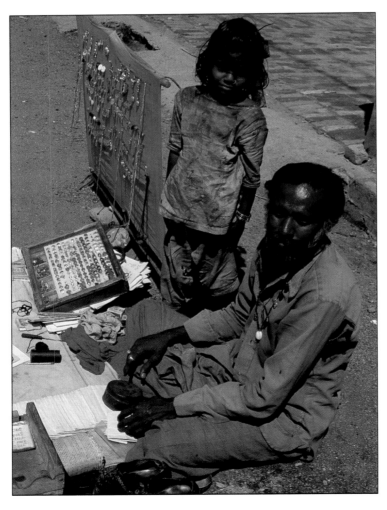

Left Parents may wonder what the future holds and how to avoid misfortune for their child. Some Hindus turn to fortune tellers to ask for guidance.

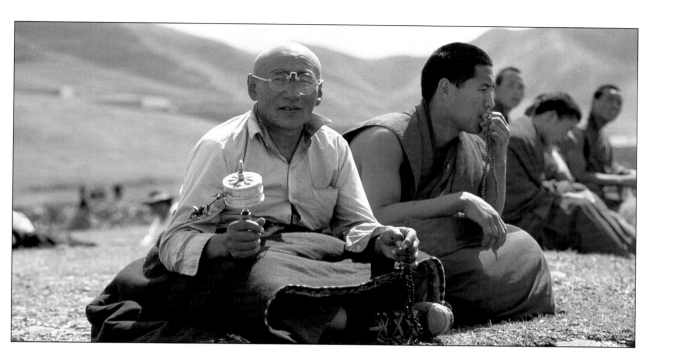

Above Buddhist monks, like these Tibetans, help people by their example, their advice and their prayers. Most Buddhists visit monasteries often to take gifts to the monks and to be helped by them.

through life. They believe their religion gives them signposts to follow and tells them how to live their lives. They have holy books to read. Many of them also believe they can discover the answers to their problems when they pray or meditate. Most religions have leaders, or groups of people, who spend their whole lives helping others to live according to their faith. Muslims have imams, Jews have rabbis, Christians have priests and ministers and Buddhists have monks.

When people believe there is a good path to follow, they want to help a baby set out in the right direction. Most parents take their baby to their religious leader, or welcome the leader to their home for prayers and blessings.

A Muslim baby is welcomed into the world with the words of the *Adhan* (Call to Prayer). This is called from the tower of a mosque five times a day when it is time for Muslims to pray.

'Allah is the greatest. I bear witness that there is no God but Allah. I bear witness that Muhammad is the messenger of Allah. Hurry to prayer. Hurry to success. Allah is the greatest.'

These words are whispered into the baby's right ear by the father or the imam. Then another prayer, which is almost the same, is whispered into the baby's left ear. From that moment the baby is a Muslim. Of course it does not yet understand the words, but the parents can feel that they have set it on the right path. As they grow older, Muslim children are taught to read the Qur'an in Arabic.

Sometimes when a Christian baby is baptized, a candle is lit and the priest or minister gives it to one of the godparents, saying:

'This is to show that you have passed from darkness to light. Shine as a light in the world to the glory of God the Father.'

This indicates that the baby should be like a light to help others. The candle is also a symbol for Jesus, the 'light' that will help the child find its way.

Orthodox Christians add another ceremony to a baptism. This is called

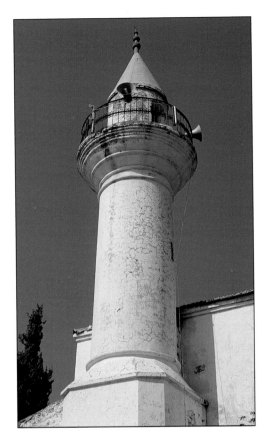

Above Muslims hear the Call to Prayer (*Adhan*) every day from the tower of the mosque. The words of the *Adhan* should also be the first words a new-born baby hears.

Chrismation. The baby's forehead, nostrils, mouth, ears and chest are all marked with crosses of holy oil. This prepares the child for life, and gives protection and strength. The oil stands for the Holy Spirit, the part of God which Christians believe is inside people, helping them to live their lives.

For Hindus the path of life begins even before a person is born. There are a number of steps along the path which are marked by ceremonies. These are called *samskaras*. There are sixteen altogether. Three happen while the mother is expecting the baby. The fourth *samskara* is when the special word *AUM* is written on the baby's tongue. Then, ten days after the birth the baby is named, at the fifth *samskara*. The sixth *samskara* is when the baby is taken outside to see the sun for the first time. The seventh is when it is given its first solid food. The eighth ceremony takes place when the baby's ears are pierced and the ninth is when all its hair is shaved off around its first birthday. There is another important *samskara* when the child is aged about seven.

All of these ceremonies take place in front of a special little fire. More than half of the sixteen ceremonies take place before the child's first birthday. This is to make sure that it is on the right path from the beginning.

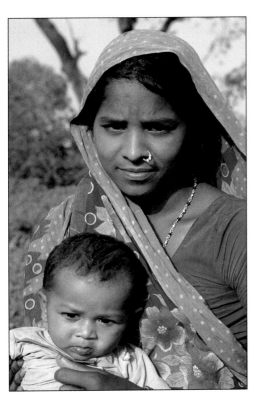

Below This baby has been through seven of the sixteen ceremonies which mark a Hindu child's path through life.

Glossary

Ancestors   People far back in a family's history.

Baptize   To sprinkle a person with water, or immerse him or her in water, as a sign that he or she is cleansed from sin, and accepted as a member of the Christian Church.

Ceremony   A formal act, often carried out as part of a custom.

Christened   Given a Christian name in a baptism service.

Circumcise   To remove the fold of skin covering the tip of a boy's penis.

Confirmation   A ceremony in the Christian church in which a person confirms his or her faith in the church.

Devil   The chief spirit of evil and enemy of God, often seen as the ruler of hell.

Eternal   Lasting for ever.

Faiths   Specific systems of religious beliefs.

Gurdwara   A Sikh place of worship.

Imam   A Muslim who leads the prayers in a mosque.

Incense   A substance that is burned to produce a sweet smell.

Meditation   Thinking deeply about something.

Monks   Male members of a religious community, who promise to be poor, obedient and pure.

Nirvana   Final release from being reborn over and over again. This is reached when a person no longer has any selfish desires.

Orthodox Christians   Members of the division of the Christian church mainly based in Eastern Europe.

Orthodox Judaism   The form of Judaism that strictly follows the teachings of Moses.

Penis   The male sex organ.

Soul   The spirit of a person. Some people believe it survives the body after death.

Symbolize   To represent or stand for something else.

Torah   The book of the teachings of Moses that forms part of the basis of Jewish teaching.

Zakat   The rule that Muslims should give 2.5% of their income and certain kinds of property to charity.

Further information

Books to read

The following series cover many aspects of different religions, including birth customs:

My Belief   (Franklin Watts, 1989)
Our Culture   (Franklin Watts, 1989)
Religions of the World   (Simon & Schuster, 1992)
Religions of the World   (Wayland, 1986)
Religious Topics   (Wayland, 1987)

Classroom materials:

A Gift to the Child   Religious Education in the Early Years Project, University of Birmingham, School of Education (Simon & Schuster, 1991) This useful pack contains a teacher's source book, pupils' books and a cassette.

Picture acknowledgements

The publishers wish to thank the following for supplying the photographs in this book: J Allan Cash 5 (top), 28, 29; Cephas Picture Library 7, 15, 20 (all Nigel Blythe); Chapel Studios 22 (Zul Mukhida); Bruce Coleman Ltd 14 (Kenneth Fischer); Eye Ubiquitous 12 (Julia Waterlow); Sonia Halliday 5 (bottom); Hutchison Picture Library 4 (Christine Pemberton), 8, 9 (Nancy Durrell McKenna) 11, 18, 19 (top, Nancy Durrell McKenna), 19 (bottom, Liba Taylor), 21, 25 (both Liba Taylor); Icorec 6; Images of India 10 (Roderick Johnson); Wayland Picture Library 16, 17 (Julia Waterlow), 23, 24 (David Cumming), 26, 27 (Richard Sharpley).

Index

Numbers in **bold** indicate photographs

291 vR